C000104019

SOUS VIDE
Vegan COOKBOOK

THE EASY FOOLPROOF TECHNIQUE TO COOK
HEALTHY RECIPES. PERFECT FOR EVERYONE,
FROM BEGINNER TO ADVANCED.

Sophia Marchesi

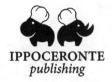

IPPOCERONTE
publishing

CONTENTS

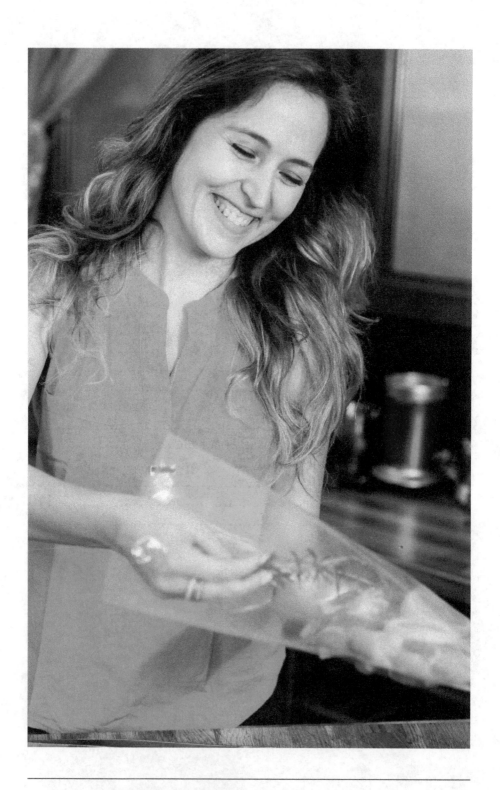

INTRODUCTION

Cooking is something that runs in my blood, most of my food memories are of my Nan cooking Sunday dinners - lasagna and cannelloni to share with the whole family. When I was young I've never liked to be stuck in a classroom, I started culinary school at a very young age, and the only thing I really wanted was to be out cooking. You could say I wasn't a very good student but I have always been really passionate about food.

I have been working in a professional kitchen since I was seventeen years old and I'm running my own restaurant since I was 23. The past thirty years have been a rewarding, yet arduous journey that I spent learning the basics and mastering the different cuisines and techniques by taking the best out of each of them. It was last year, during the lockdown, that I realized that I was starting to lose my passion. Preparing a dish had become an aseptic and mechanical where perfection was king.

I wanted to go back to my roots, cooking has always been about my family; preparing a dish together with the people I love gives me time to connect and create precious memories. Setting aside a time where the entire family can work together to create a meal gives us a chance to pause, catch up and just connect with each other.

What I would like to share with you in this book is my renewed passion and a technique that I learned during my time in France, the Sous Vide. This innovative cooking method is something my grandmother never thought existed and creates the perfect opportunity to spend some time in the kitchen with my family. For these reasons, I think the Sous Vide is the perfect combination of my professional and domestic life.

Sous Vide is the French term that translates to "under vacuum" and it is the method for preparing a dish at a specifically controlled temperature and time; your food should be prepared at the temperature at which it will be eaten. Put simply, this procedure involves placing food in vacuum seal bags and boiling it in a specially-built bath of water for longer than average cooking times (usually 1 to 7 hours, up to 48 or more in some cases). Cooking at an exact temperature takes the guesswork out of the equation that defines a perfect meal. You can easily prepare your steak, chicken, lamb, pork, etc., exactly the way you like it, every single time.

It's easy to use and leads to great results every time. You'll end up with food that's more tender and juicier than anything else you've ever made. This technique will help you to take your everyday cooking to a higher level. To do a top dish, most of the time, you don't need exotic ingredients, it is just a matter to get the best from the ingredients you already know.

The greatest part of Sous Vide cooking is that it does not require your constant presence in the kitchen. When the food is sealed in a bag and placed in the water bath, you can leave it at a low temperature, and it will cook on its own without asking much of your attention. The Sous Vide Cookers that are nowadays available in the market are efficient at regulating the perfect temperature to cook food according to its texture while maintaining the minimum required temperature. So, while your food is in the water, your hands are practically free to work on other important tasks or spend some quality time with your family.

It is an artful skill that is definitely worth trying. If it is just your first time, don't feel bad if you don't get the results you wanted to achieve. You will get better by gaining experience with this cookbook! The key is having patience, the right information, and consistency.

The meals prepared with Sous Vide are tasty and healthy, since this technique does not use added fats during the preparation of your dish also, using low temperature ensures that the perfect cooking point is reached.

Dishes included in this cookbook are simple, delicious, and provide you with so many options that you'll be preparing them for years to come. These recipes are made to be shared with the people you love and to build new precious food memories as I did with my Nan.

RECIPES

1. FENNEL PICKLE WITH LEMON

Cal.: 156 | Fat: 5g | Protein: 1g

Preparation Time: 31 minutes
Cooking Time: 30 minutes
Servings: 5

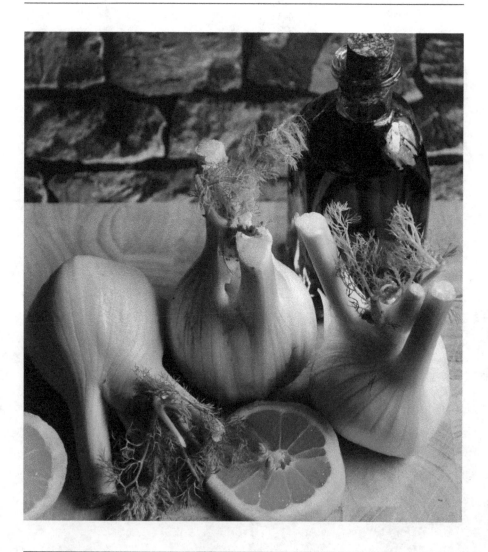

Ingredients

1 cup white wine vinegar
2 tablespoons beet sugar
Juice and zest from 1 lemon
1 teaspoon kosher salt
2 medium bulb fennels trimmed up and cut into ¼
inch thick slices.

Directions

1. Prepare the water bath using your immersion circulator and raise the temperature to 180°F/82°C.

2. Take a large bowl and add the vinegar, sugar, lemon juice, salt, lemon zest and whisk them well.

3. Transfer the mixture to your resealable zip bag.

4. Add the fennel and seal using the immersion method.

5. Immerse underwater and cook for 30 minutes.

6. Transfer to an ice bath and allow the mixture to reach the room temperature.

7. Serve!

2. BUDDHA'S DELIGHT

Cal.: 186 | Fat: 10g | Protein: 6g

Preparation Time: 21 minutes
Cooking Time: 1 hour
Servings: 8

Ingredients

1 cup vegetable broth
2 tablespoons tomato paste
1 tablespoon grated ginger
1 tablespoon rice wine
1 tablespoon rice wine vinegar
1 tablespoon agave nectar
2 teaspoons Sriracha sauce
3 minced garlic cloves
2 boxes of cubed tofu

Directions

1. Prepare your water bath using your immersion circulator and raise the temperature to 185°F/85°C.

2. Take a medium bowl and add all the listed ingredients except the tofu.

3. Mix well.

---

4. Transfer the mixture to a heavy-duty resealable zipper bag and top with the tofu.

5. Seal it up using the immersion method. Cook for 1 hour.

6. Pour the contents into a serving bowl

7. Serve!

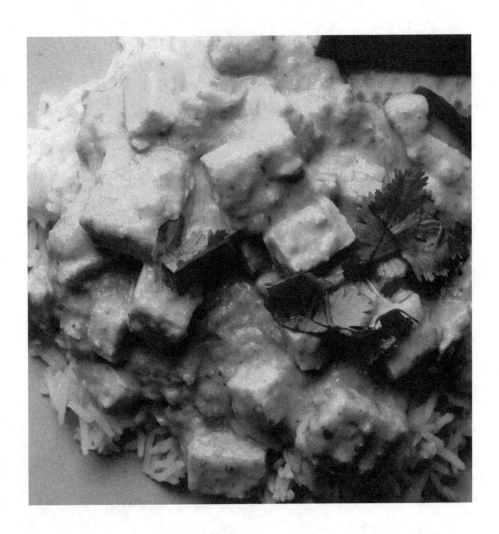

3. ITALIAN PICKLED VEGETABLES

Cal.: 245 | Fat: 4g | Protein: 7g

Preparation Time: 31 minutes
Cooking Time: 1 hour
Servings: 8

Ingredients

2 cups white wine vinegar
1 cup water
½ cup beet sugar
3 tablespoons kosher salt
1 tablespoon whole black peppercorns
1 cup cauliflower, cut up into ½-inch pieces
1 stemmed and seeded bell pepper, cut up into
½-inch pieces
1 cup carrots, cut up into ½-inch pieces
½ thinly sliced white onion
2 seeded and stemmed Serrano peppers, cut up into
½-inch pieces

Directions

1. Prepare the sous-vide water bath using your immersion circulator and raise the temperature to 180°F/82°C.

---

2. Take a large bowl and mix in vinegar, sugar, salt, water and peppercorns.

3. Transfer the mixture to a large resealable zipper bag and add the cauliflower, onion, serrano peppers, vinegar mixture, bell pepper, and carrots.

4. Seal it up using the immersion method and immerse underwater, cook for about 1 hour.

5. Once cooked, take it out from the bag and serve

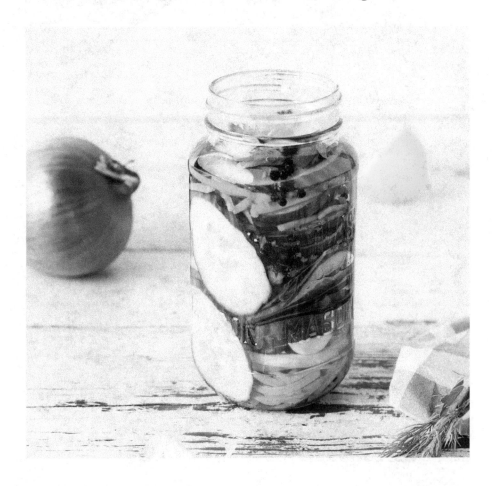

4. VEGAN STEEL CUT OATS

Cal.: 344 | Fat: 21g | Protein: 19g

Preparation Time: 3 hours and 20 minutes
Cooking Time: 3 minutes
Servings: 5

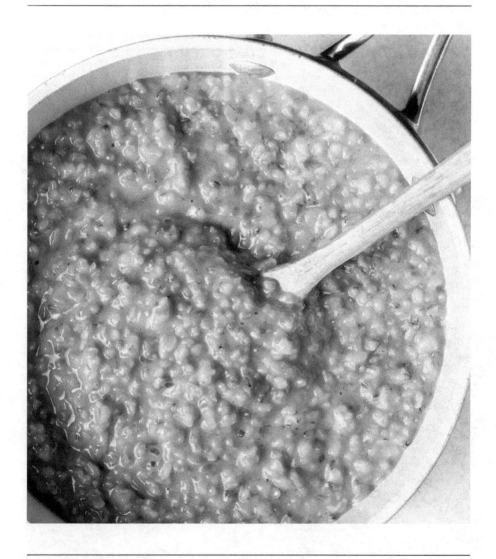

Ingredients

2 cups water
½ cup steel cut oats
½ teaspoon salt
Cinnamon and maple syrup for topping

Directions

1. Prepare the water bath by using your immersion circulator and raise the temperature to 180°F/82°C.

2. Take a heavy-duty resealable zipper bag and add all the listed ingredients except the cinnamon and maple syrup.

3. Seal the bag using the immersion method and Immerse underwater.

4. Cook for about 3 hours.

5. Once cooked, remove it, and transfer the oats to your serving bowl.

6. Serve with a sprinkle of cinnamon and some maple syrup.

5. HONEY ROASTED CARROTS

Cal.: 174 | Fat: 2g | Protein: 1g

Preparation Time: 6 minutes
Cooking Time: 75 minutes
Servings: 4

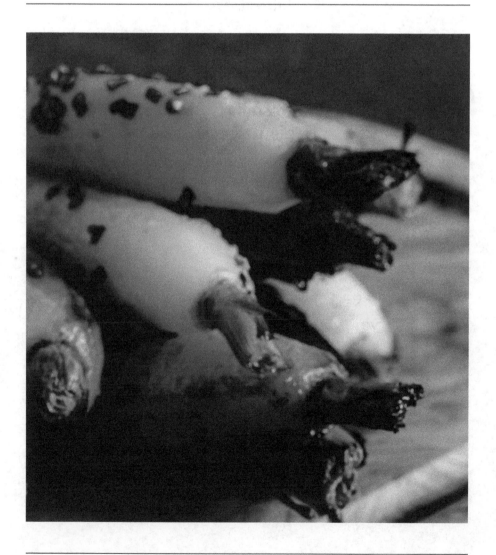

Ingredients

1-pound baby carrots
4 tablespoons vegan butter
3 tablespoons honey
¼ teaspoon kosher salt
¼ teaspoon ground cardamom

Directions

1. Prepare the sous-vide water bath using your immersion circulator and increase the temperature to 185°F/85°C.

2. Add the carrots, honey, whole butter, kosher salt, and cardamom to a resealable bag.

3. Seal using the immersion method. Cook for 75 minutes and once done, remove it from the water bath.

4. Strain the glaze by passing through a fine mesh.

5. Set it aside.

6. Take the carrots out from the bag and pour any excess glaze over them. Serve with a few seasonings.

6. GARLIC CITRUS ARTICHOKES

Cal.: 408 | Fat: 12g | Protein: 20g

Preparation Time: 31 minutes
Cooking Time: 90 minutes
Servings: 4

Ingredients

4 tablespoons freshly squeezed lemon juice
12 pieces' baby artichokes
4 tablespoons vegan butter
2 fresh garlic cloves, minced.
1 teaspoon fresh lemon zest
Kosher salt, and black pepper, to taste
Chopped up fresh parsley for garnishing.

Directions

1. Prepare the water bath using your immersion circulator and raise the temperature to 180°F/82°C.

2. Take a large bowl and add the cold water and 2 tablespoons of lemon juice.

3. Peel and discard the outer tough layer of your artichoke and cut them into quarters.

---

4. Transfer to a cold-water bath and let it sit for a while.

5. Take a large skillet and put it over medium-high heat.

6. Add in the butter to the skillet and allow the butter to melt.

7. Add the garlic alongside 2 tablespoons of lemon juice and the zest.

8. Remove from heat and season with a bit of pepper and salt.

9. Allow it to cool for about 5 minutes.

10. Then, drain the artichokes from the cold water and place them in a large resealable bag. Add in the butter mixture as well.

11. Seal it up using the immersion method and immerse underwater for about 1 and a ½ hour.

12. Once cooked, transfer the artichokes to a bowl and serve with a garnish of parsley.

7. HONEY TRUFFLE SUNCHOKES

Cal.: 255 | Fat: 5g | Protein: 10g

Preparation Time: 16 minutes
Cooking Time: 90 minutes
Servings: 4

Ingredients

8 ounces peeled Sunchokes, sliced into ¼ inch thick
pieces
3 tablespoons unsalted vegan butter
2 tablespoons agave nectar
1 teaspoon truffle oil
Kosher salt, and black pepper, to taste

Directions

1. Prepare the water bath using your immersion circulator and raise the temperature to 180°F/82°C.

2. Take a heavy-duty resealable zip bag and add the butter, nectar, sunchokes and truffle oil and mix them well.

3. Sprinkle some salt and pepper, and then seal using the immersion method.

4. Immerse it underwater and cook for 1 ½ hour.

5. Once cooked, transfer the contents to a skillet.

6. Put the skillet over medium-high heat and cook for 5 minutes more until the liquid has evaporated.

7. Season with pepper and salt to adjust the flavor if needed

8. Serve!

8. VEGAN CAULIFLOWER ALFREDO

Cal.: 160 | Fat: 8g | Protein: 11g

Preparation Time: 16 minutes
Cooking Time: 90 minutes
Servings: 6

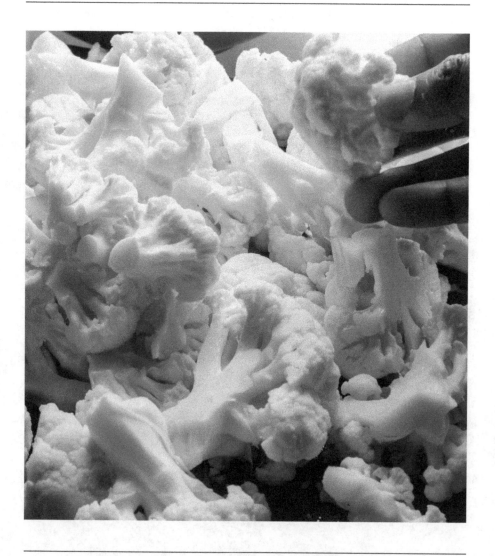

Ingredients

4 cups chopped cauliflower.
2 cups water
2/3 cup cashews
2 garlic cloves
½ teaspoon dried oregano
½ teaspoon dried basil
½ teaspoon dried rosemary
4 tablespoons nutritional yeast
Salt, and pepper to taste

Directions

1. Prepare the sous-vide water bath using your immersion circulator and increase the temperature to 170°F/76°C.

2. Take a heavy-duty resealable zip bag and add the cashews, cauliflower, oregano, water, garlic, rosemary and basil.

3. Seal using the immersion method. Immerse underwater and cook for 90 minutes.

4. Transfer the cooked contents to a blender and purée.

5. Use Alfredo over your favorite pasta.

9. MARINATED MUSHROOMS

Cal.: 440 | Fat: 19g | Protein: 28g

Preparation Time: 21 minutes
Cooking Time: 1 hour
Servings: 2

Ingredients

10 large button mushrooms
3 tablespoons truffle oil
3 tablespoons olive oil
1 tablespoon chopped fresh thyme.
1 thinly sliced garlic clove
Salt, and pepper to taste

Directions

1. Prepare the sous-vide water bath using your immersion circulator and raise the temperature to 185°F/85°C.

2. Take a large bowl and add the truffle oil, mushrooms, olive oil, garlic, and thyme.

3. Season with some pepper and salt.

4. Transfer the mushroom mixture to a large sous-vide resealable zip bag and add the mixture to the bag.

---

5. Seal it up using the immersion method. Immerse underwater and cook for 1 hour.

6. Once cooked, drain the mushrooms, and discard the cooking liquid.

7. Take a large skillet and put it over medium heat for 3 minutes.

8. Add the mushrooms and sear for about 1 minute to brown it.

9. Transfer the cooked mushroom to a serving plate and season with pepper and salt.

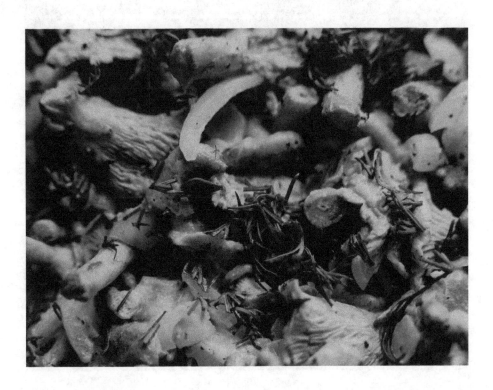

10. CANNELLINIBEANSWITHHERBS

Cal.: 578 | Fat: 31g | Protein: 18g

Preparation Time: 16 minutes
Cooking Time: 3 hours
Servings: 5

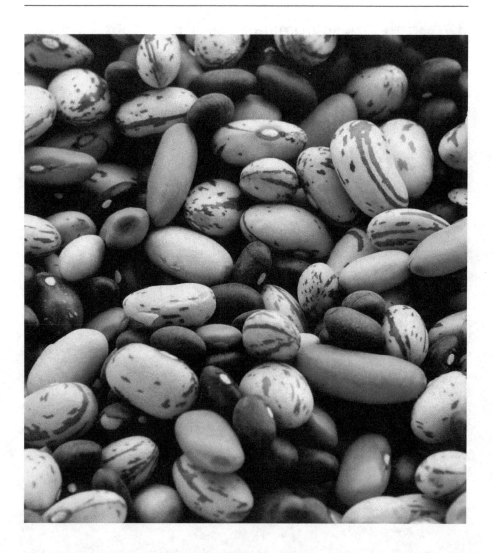

Ingredients

1 cup cannellini beans (dried) soaked overnight in
salty cold water.
1 cup water
½ cup extra-virgin olive oil
1 peeled carrot, cut up into 1-inch dice.
1 celery stalk, cut up into 1-inch dice.
1 quartered shallot
4 crushed garlic cloves
2 fresh rosemary sprigs
2 bay leaves
Kosher salt, and pepper to taste

Directions

1. Prepare the water bath using your sous-vide immersion circulator and raise the temperature to 190°F/88°C.

2. Drain the soaked beans and rinse them.

3. Transfer to a heavy-duty resealable zip bag and add the olive oil, celery, water, carrot, shallot, garlic, rosemary and bay leaves. Season with pepper and salt.

4. Seal using the immersion method and cook for 3 hours.

5. Once cooked, remove the beans and check for seasoning. Discard the rosemary and serve!

11. NAVY BEANS

Cal.: 210 | Fat: 14g | Protein: 2g

Preparation Time: 15 minutes
Cooking Time: 3 hours
Servings: 8

Ingredients

1 cup dried and soaked navy beans
1 cup water
½ cup extra-virgin olive oil
1 peeled carrot, cut up into 1-inch dices
1 stalk celery, cut up into 1-inch dices
1 quartered shallot
4 cloves crushed garlic
2 sprigs of fresh rosemary
2 pieces' bay leaves
Kosher salt, to taste
Freshly ground black pepper, to taste

Directions

1. Prepare your sous-vide water bath using your immersion circulator and raise the temperature to 190°F/88°C.

---

2. Carefully drain and rinse your beans and add them alongside the rest of the ingredients to a heavy-duty zip bag.

3. Seal using the immersion method and immerse it underwater. Cook for about 3 hours.

4. Once cooked, taste the beans.

5. If they are firm, then cook for another 1 hour and pour them in a serving bowl.

6. Serve!

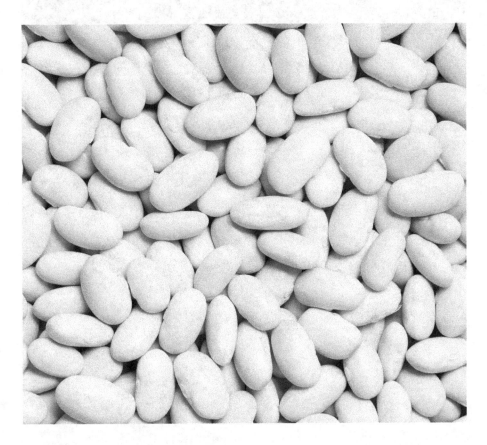

12. BUTTERED RADISHES

Cal.: 134 | Fat: 1g | Protein: 0.3g

Preparation Time: 6 minutes
Cooking Time: 46 minutes
Servings: 4

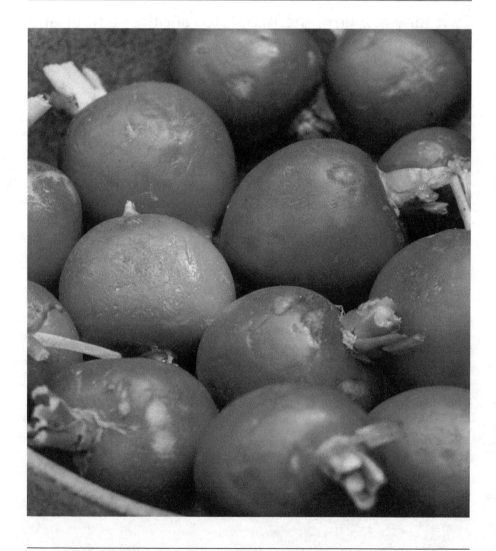

Ingredients

1-pound radishes, cut up in half lengthwise
3 tablespoons vegan butter
½ teaspoon sea salt

Directions

1. Prepare your water bath using your immersion circulator and raise the temperature to 190°F/88°C.

2. Add your radish halves, butter and salt in a resealable zipper bag and seal it up using the immersion method.

3. Immerse underwater and cook for 45 minutes.

4. Once cooked, strain the liquid and discard.

5. Serve the radishes in a bowl!

13. RHUBARB

Cal.: 111 | Fat: 1g | Protein: 0.2g

Preparation Time: 16 minutes
Cooking Time: 40 minutes
Servings: 4

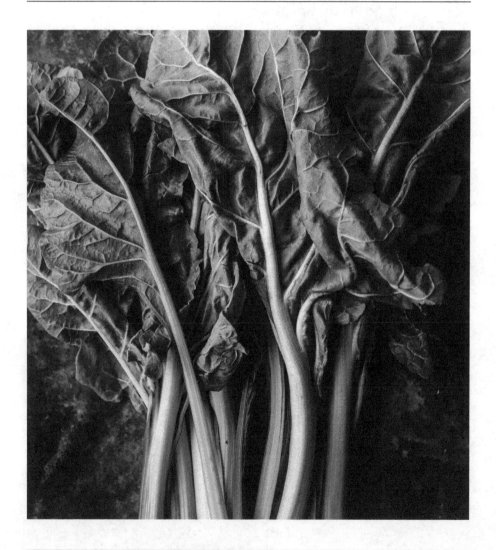

Ingredients

2 cups rhubarb
1 tablespoon Grand Marnier
1 teaspoon beet sugar
½ teaspoon kosher salt
½ a teaspoon freshly ground black pepper

Directions

1. Prepare the sous-vide water bath to a temperature of 140°F/60°C. using your immersion circulator.

2. Take a large heavy-duty resealable zip bag and add all the listed ingredients. Whisk everything well.

3. Seal the bag using the immersion method/water displacement method.

4. Place it under your preheated water and cook for about 40 minutes.

5. Once cooked, take the bag out from the water bath, take the contents out and place it on a serving plate.

6. Serve warm!

14. CHINESE BLACK BEAN SAUCE

Cal.: 375 | Fat: 12g | Protein: 12g

Preparation Time: 21 minutes
Cooking Time: 90 minutes
Servings: 4

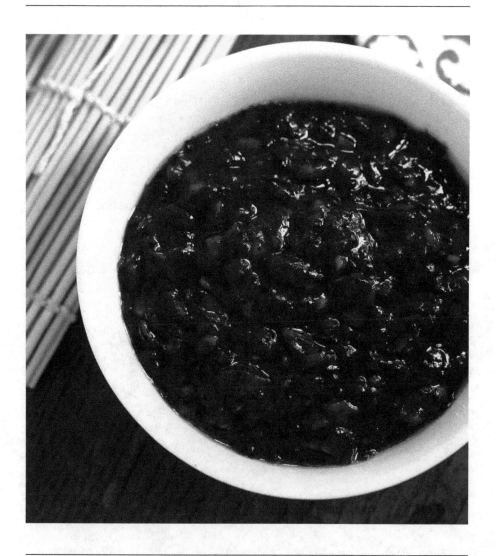

Ingredients

4 cups halved green beans.
3 minced garlic cloves
2 teaspoons rice wine vinegar
1½ tablespoons prepared black bean sauce.
1 tablespoon olive oil

Directions

1. Prepare the sous-vide water bath using your immersion circulator and raise the temperature to 170°F/76°C.

2. Add all the listed ingredients into a large mixing bowl alongside the green beans. Coat everything evenly.

3. Take a heavy-duty zip bag and add the mixture.

4. Zip the bag using the immersion method and immerse it underwater.

5. Cook for about 1 hour and 30 minutes.

6. Once cooked, take it out and serve immediately!

15. CHIPOTLE AND BLACK BEANS

Cal.: 466 | Fat: 20g | Protein: 37g

Preparation Time: 21 minutes
Cooking Time: 6 hours
Servings: 6

Ingredients

1 cup dry black beans
2 2/3 cup water
1/3 cup freshly squeezed orange juice
2 tablespoons orange zest
1 teaspoon salt
1 teaspoon cumin
½ teaspoon chipotle chili powder

Directions

1. Prepare the sous-vide water bath using your immersion circulator and raise the temperature to 170°F/76°C.

2. Add all the listed ingredients into a large mixing bowl alongside the green beans. Coat everything evenly.

3. Take a heavy-duty zip bag and add the mixture.

4. Zip the bag using the immersion method and immerse it underwater.

5. Cook for about 1 hour and 30 minutes.

6. Once cooked, take it out and serve immediately!

16. PICKLED MIXED VEGGIES

Cal.: 174 | Fat: 4g | Protein: 2g

Preparation Time: 11 minutes
Cooking Time: 40 minutes
Servings: 4

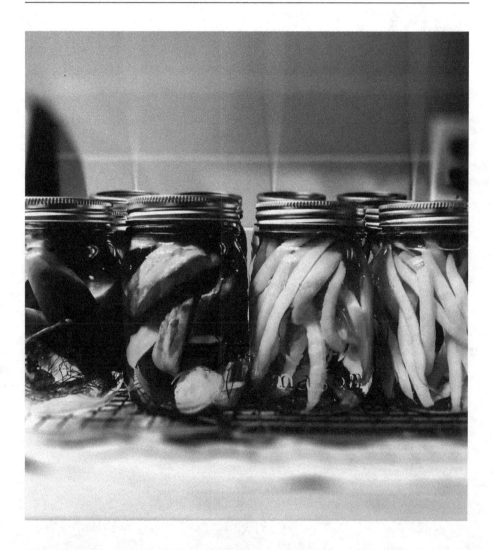

Ingredients

12 oz. beets, cut up into ½-inch slices
½ Serrano pepper, seeds removed
1 garlic clove, diced
2/3 cup white vinegar
2/3 cup filtered water
2 tablespoons pickling spice

Directions

1. Prepare the sous-vide water bath using your immersion circulator and raise the temperature to 190°F/88°C.

2. Take 4–6 ounces' mason jar and add the Serrano pepper, beets and garlic cloves.

3. Take a medium stock pot and add the pickling spice, filtered water, white vinegar and bring the mixture to a boil.

4. Remove the stock and strain the mix over the

5. beets in the jar.

6. Fill them up.

7. Seal it loosely and immerse it underwater. Cook for 40 minutes.

8. Allow the jars to cool and serve!

17. ROOT VEGETABLES MIX

Cal.: 268 | Fat: 6g | Protein: 10g

Preparation Time: 15 minutes
Cooking Time: 3 hours
Servings: 4

Ingredients

1 peeled turnip, cut up into 1-inch pieces
1 peeled rutabaga, cut up into 1-inch pieces
8 pieces petite carrots peeled up and cut into 1-inch pieces
1 peeled parsnip, cut up into 1-inch pieces
½ red onion, cut up into 1-inch pieces and peeled
4 pieces' garlic, crushed
4 sprigs of fresh rosemary
2 tablespoons extra-virgin olive oil
Kosher salt, and black pepper to taste
2 tablespoons unsalted vegan butter

Directions

1. Prepare the sous-vide water bath using your immersion circulator and raise the temperature to 185°F/85°C.

---

2. Take two large heavy-duty resealable zipper bags and divide the vegetables and the rosemary between the bags.

3. Add 1 tablespoon oil to the bag and season with some salt and pepper.

4. Seal the bags using the immersion method. Immerse underwater and cook for 3 hours.

5. Take a skillet and place it over high heat and add in the oil.

6. Once done, add the contents of your bag to the skillet. Cook the mixture for about 5–6 minutes until the liquid comes to a syrupy consistency.

7. Add the butter to your veggies and toss them well.

8. Keep cooking for another 5 minutes until they are nicely browned. Serve!

18. PICKLED CARROTS

Cal.: 127 | Fat: 2g | Protein: 1g

Preparation Time: 31 minutes
Cooking Time: 90 minutes
Servings: 1

Ingredients

1 cup white wine vinegar
½ cup beet sugar
3 tablespoons kosher salt
1 teaspoon black peppercorns
1/3 cup ice-cold water
10–12 pieces' petite carrots, peeled with the stems trimmed
4 sprigs of fresh thyme
2 peeled garlic cloves

Directions

1. Prepare the sous-vide water bath using your immersion circulator and raise the temperature to 190°F/88°C.

2. Take a medium-sized saucepan and add the vinegar, salt, sugar and peppercorns and place it over medium heat.

---

3. Then, let the mixture reach the boiling point and keep stirring until the sugar has dissolved alongside the salt

4. Remove the heat and add the cold water.

5. Allow the mixture to cool down to room temperature.

6. Take a resealable bag and add the thyme, carrots and garlic alongside the brine solution and seal it up using the immersion method.

7. Immerse underwater and cook for 90 minutes.

8. Once cooked, remove the bag from the water bath and place into an ice bath.

9. Carefully take the carrots out from the bag and serve.

19. GARLIC TOMATOES

Cal.: 289 | Fat: 11g | Protein: 8g

Preparation Time: 11 minutes
Cooking Time: 45 minutes
Servings: 4

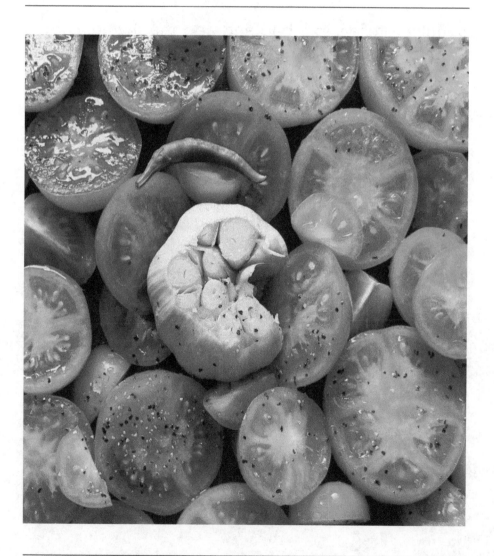

Ingredients

4 pieces cored and diced tomatoes.
2 tablespoons extra-virgin olive oil
3 minced garlic cloves
1 teaspoon dried oregano
1 teaspoon fine sea salt

Directions

1. Prepare the sous-vide water bath using your immersion circulator and raise the temperature to 145°F/63°C.

2. Add all the listed ingredients to the resealable bag and seal using the immersion method.

3. Immerse underwater and let it cook for 45 minutes.

4. Once cooked, transfer the tomatoes to a serving plate.

5. Serve with some vegan French bread slices.

20. SWEET CURRIED WINTER SQUASH

Cal.: 185 | Fat: 2g | Protein: 9g

Preparation Time: 21 minutes
Cooking Time: 1 hour 30 minutes
Servings: 6

Ingredients

1 medium winter squash
2 tablespoons unsalted vegan butter
1 to 2 tablespoons Thai curry paste
½ teaspoon kosher salt
Fresh cilantro for serving.
Lime wedges for serving.

Directions

1. Prepare the sous-vide water bath using your immersion circulator and raise the temperature to 185°F/85°C.

2. Slice up the squash into half lengthwise and scoop out the seeds alongside the inner membrane. Keep the seeds for later use.

3. Slice the squash into wedges of about 1 ½-inch thickness.

---

4. Take a large heavy-duty bag resealable zip bag and add the squash wedges, curry paste, butter and salt and seal it using the immersion method.

5. Immerse it underwater and let it cook for 1 ½ hour.

6. Once cooked, remove the bag from water and give it a slight squeeze until it is soft.

7. If it is not soft, then add to the water once again and cook for 40 minutes more.

8. Transfer the cooked dish to a serving plate and drizzle with a bit of curry butter sauce from the bag.

9. Top your squash with a bit of cilantro, lime wedges and serve!

21. VEGAN CAULIFLOWER ALFREDO WITH CASHEWS

Cal.: 350 | Fat: 20g | Protein: 9g

Preparation Time: 9 minutes
Cooking Time: 1 hour 30 minutes
Servings: 6

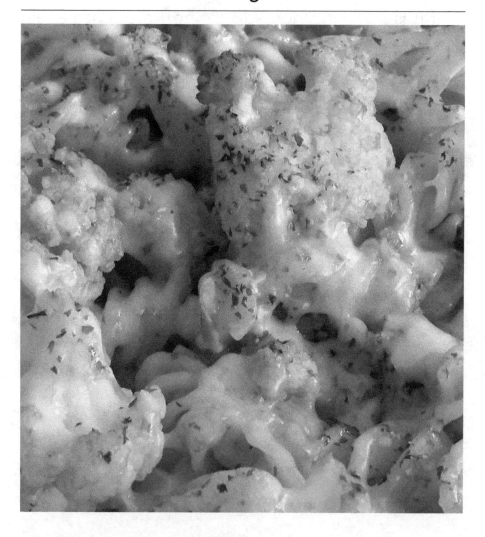

Ingredients

4 tablespoons nutritional yeast
Salt and pepper
½ teaspoon dried rosemary
4 cups chopped cauliflower.
½ teaspoon dried oregano
½ teaspoon dried basil
2 garlic cloves
2 cups water
¼ cup cashews

Directions

1. Level the Sous Vide Machine to 185°F/85°C.

2. Transfer the cauliflower, liquid cashews, cloves, oregano, herbs and rosemary to a thick plastic-seal bag and cover.

3. Place the bag in the vacuum and cook for 1½ hours.

4. In a bowl, add in the contents. Mix and serve on the top of your favorite pasta.

22. VEGAN CARROT-CURRY SOUP

Cal.: 322 | Fat: 12g | Protein: 6g

Preparation Time: 9 minutes
Cooking Time: 1 hour 45 minutes
Servings: 4

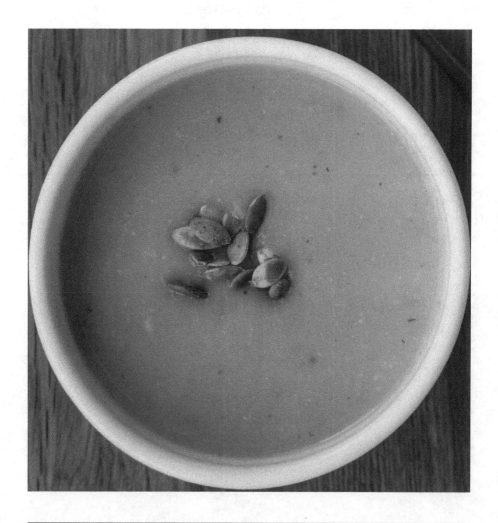

Ingredients

1 garlic clove, minced
1-pound carrots, peeled and sliced
2 teaspoons yellow curry powder
1 teaspoon ground turmeric
1 stalk lemongrass, sliced
1 cup unsweetened coconut milk
1 tablespoon Thai red chili paste
1 shallot, thinly sliced
2 teaspoons kosher salt

Directions

1. Adjust the Sous Vide Machine to 190°F/88°C.

2. In a big zipper-lock package, combine all the ingredients.

3. Use the water immersion method to close the bag and put it in the water bath. For 1 hour and 45 minutes, adjust the clock.

4. Remove the pack from the boiling water when the effects go off.

5. Discard bits of lemongrass. Move the contents of the package to a processor and purée for around 2 minutes, until smooth.

6. To achieve the desired consistency, add extra coconut milk or water. Sprinkle with salt.

23. CRUNCHY BALSAMIC ONIONS

Cal.: 757 | Fat: 29g | Protein: 13g

Preparation Time: 6 minutes
Cooking Time: 2 hours
Servings: 10

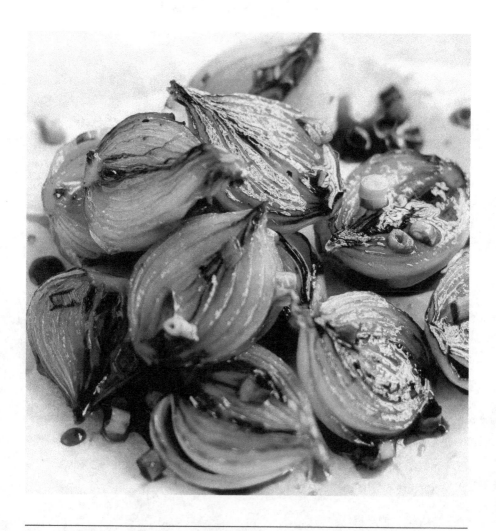

Ingredients

2 tbsp. brown sugar
Salt and pepper
2 brown onions (julienned)
1 tbsp. balsamic vinegar
2 tbsp. olive oil

Directions

1. In a jar, combine all of the components, lock and cook for 2 hours at 185°F/85°C.

2. For 3 hours or night, move to a jar and chill in the fridge.

24. VEGETABLE STOCK

Cal.: 335 | Fat: 31g | Protein: 19g

Preparation Time: 11 minutes
Cooking Time: 13 hours
Servings: 12

Ingredients

1 tablespoon whole black peppercorns
2 bay leaves
2 cups (diced) carrots.
2 cups white button mushrooms
1 bunch parsley
2 tablespoons (extra-virgin) olive oil
8 cups of water
1 cup (chopped) fennel.
6 garlic cloves (crushed)
2 cups (chopped) celery.
2 cups (chopped) leeks.

Directions

1. Adjust the Sous Vide Machine to 180°F/82°C. Heat the boiler to 450°F/230°C.

2. Toss the olive oil with the carrot, leeks, celery, fen-

nel and cloves in a large bowl.

3. Switch to a baking tray and roast for about 20 minutes, until lightly browned.

4. Move to a whole zipper-locking bag with steamed veggies, any leftover juices and golden-brown parts.

5. Add water, coriander, peppercorns, mushroom and bay leaves.

6. Close the package using the method of water immersion.

7. Place the package and press the button for 12 hours in the boiling water.

8. To prevent water evaporation, protect the water bath with plastic wrap.

9. To keep the veggies covered, apply water occasionally.

25. TURMERIC TOFU WITH SUMAC AND LIME

Cal.: 95 | Fat: 12g | Protein: 5g

Preparation Time: 13 minutes
Cooking Time: 2 hours 45 minutes
Servings: 4

Ingredients

2 limes, cut into wedges.
Sumac, for serving.
1 package firm tofu drained and sliced.
1 teaspoon ground turmeric
1 teaspoon kosher salt
2 teaspoons freshly ground black pepper.
2 tablespoon extra-virgin olive oil
4 garlic cloves, roughly minced.

Directions

1. Put the tofu planks on a baking tray that is a wash cloth-lined.

2. Add a separate towel and a separate baking sheet to the middle.

3. To measure the tofu, put a large pot or many canned goods on it.

---

4. Leave it to stay at room temperature for thirty minutes.

5. Level the Sous Vide Machine, meanwhile, to 180°F/82°C.

6. Stir together the olive oil, cloves, pepper, turmeric and salts in a small cup.

7. In a large zipper-locking or vacuum lock package, put the tofu in a single sheet.

8. With the garlic-turmeric paste, rub all edges of the tofu.

9. Use the water immersion method or a vacuum adhesive on the wet setting to close the container.

10. In the boiling water, put the bag and set the timer for 2 hours.

11. Warm the broiler heavy for about 5 minutes until the tofu is done.

12. Remove the package from the boiling water when the timer goes off.

13. Remove the tofu carefully from the bag and put it on a baking tray lined with foil.

14. Sprinkle over the tofu with any leftover oil from the packet.

15. Roast until golden brown on either edge, 3 minutes.

16. Shift to a tray for serving. Squeeze over the tofu with lemon juice and scatter with cilantro. Serve hot.

26. TOMATO-BASIL PASTA SAUCE

Cal.: 67 | Fat: 19g | Protein: 5g

Preparation Time: 8 minutes
Cooking Time: 1 hour 15 minutes
Servings: 7

Ingredients

3 bay leaves
1 teaspoon red pepper flakes
1 can (crushed) tomatoes
1 tablespoon (extra-virgin) olive oil
1 tablespoon garlic salt
2 cups fresh basil leaves
1 carrot (peeled and finely diced)
½ white onion (finely chopped)

Directions

1. Preheat the Sous Vide machine to 185°F/85°C.

2. In a big zipper-locking package, mix all the ingredients.

3. Wrap the package using the method of water immersion.

4. Set the timer for 1 hour or up to 2 hours and put the package in the water bath.

5. Take the package from the boiling water when the timer goes off.

6. Shift the entire stock of the package to a food processor.

7. Discard the bay leaves and purée for about 30 seconds until creamy.

8. Eat with pasta. It is also possible to cool and chill in the fridge for up to 2 days or preserve for up to a month.

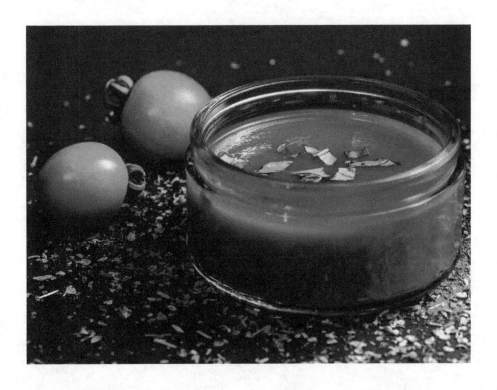

27. CONFIT GARLIC

Cal.: 105 | Fat: 18g | Protein: 6g

Preparation Time: 11 minutes
Cooking Time: 1 hour 4 hours 10 minutes
Servings: 8

Ingredients

1 tablespoon kosher salt
¼ cup (extra-virgin) olive oil
1 cup (peeled) garlic cloves

Directions

1. Level the Sous Vide Machine to 190°F/88°C.

2. In a complete zipper-locking or vacuum sealing container, mix all the ingredients.

3. Use the water immersion method or a vacuum adhesive on the wet setting to seal the container.

4. Place the package in the water bath and set a timer for 4 hours. Take the bag from the boiling water when the timer goes off.

5. Move the confit to an enclosed storage container and cool for up to one month.

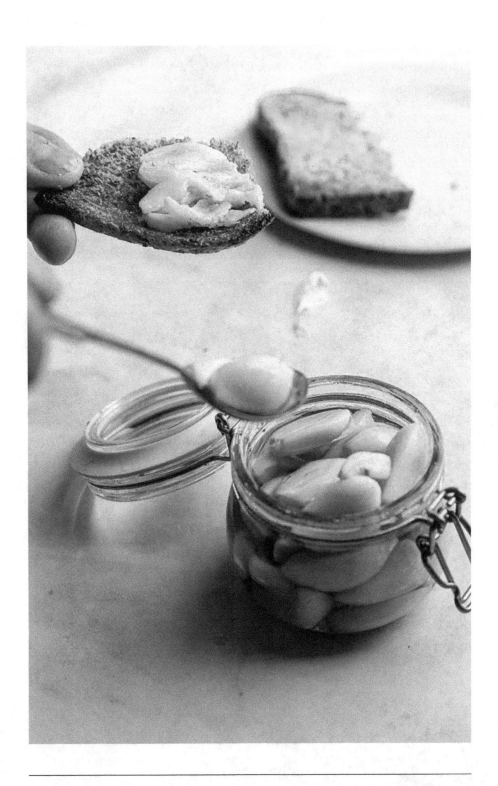

28. QUINOA

Cal.: 156 | Fat: 21g | Protein: 8g

Preparation Time: 6 minutes
Cooking Time: 1 hour 5 minutes
Servings: 6

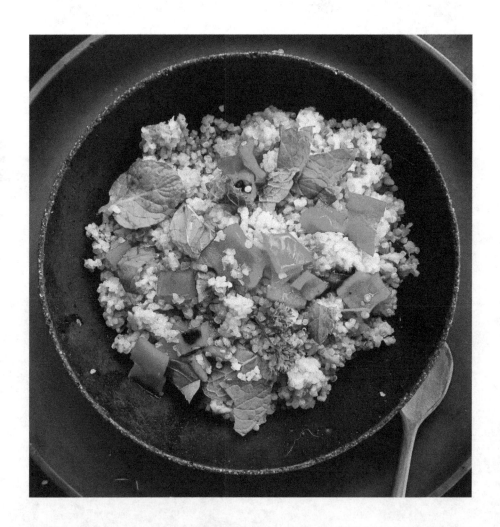

Ingredients

Kosher salt
1 ½ cups water
1 cup quinoa (rinsed)
1 small sprig of fresh basil
2 garlic cloves (peeled)

Directions

1. Adjust the Sous Vide Machine to 180°F/82°C.

2. In a complete sealed bag, mix the quinoa, cloves, basil and ½ teaspoon salt.

3. Use the water immersion method, add the water and close the package.

4. In the boiling water, put the bag then set the timer for 1 hour.

5. Remove the package from the boiling water as soon as the timer goes off.

6. To a medium cup, move the entire contents of the package and remove the basil and cloves.

7. Fluff the quinoa using a spoon and season with salt.

29. STRAWBERRY-RHUBARB JAM

Cal.: 36 | Fat: 9g | Protein: 18g

Preparation Time: 8 minutes
Cooking Time: 1 hour 45 minutes
Servings: 12

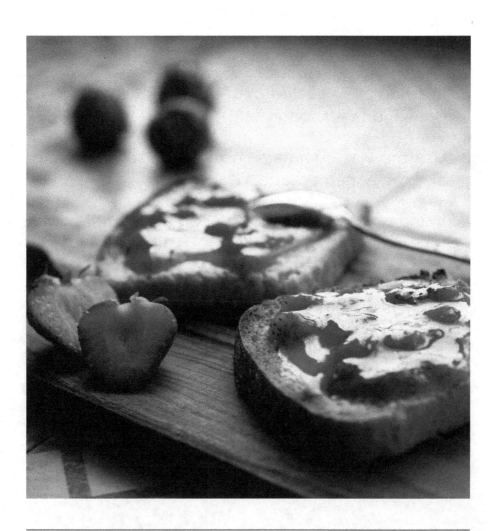

Ingredients

2 tablespoons powdered pectin
2 tablespoons (freshly squeezed) lemon juice.
1 cup granulated sugar
1 cup (diced) strawberries.
1 cup (chopped) rhubarb.

Directions

1. Level the Sous Vide Machine to 180°F/82°C.

2. In a big zipper-locking package, mix all the ingredients.

3. Use the water immersion method to close the bag and put it in the boiling water. For 2 hours, set the timer.

4. Remove the package from the boiling water when the timer goes off.

5. Move the pack's entire contents to an enclosed jar and let it cool down to room temperature. For up to 1 month, put it in the fridge.

30. SUNCHOKES WITH TOASTED MARCONI ALMONDS

Cal.: 120 | Fat: 17g | Protein: 6g

Preparation Time: 13 minutes
Cooking Time: 1 hours 40 minutes
Servings: 4

Ingredients

2 tablespoons (chopped) Marconi almonds.
(Minced) fresh chives
1 ½ pounds sunchokes (scrubbed)
4 tablespoons (extra-virgin) olive oil
Kosher salt
(freshly ground) black pepper.

Directions

1. Level the Sous Vide Machine to 194°F/90°C.

2. Put the sunchokes, salt and black pepper in a vacuum seal package or large zipper-locking.

3. Pour one tablespoon olive oil.

4. Use the water immersion method or a vacuum adhesive on the wet setting to seal the container.

5. In the boiling water, put the bag and set a timer for one hour.

6. Heat the oven to 450°F about ten minutes until the timer goes off.

7. Cover with foil on a rimmed baking dish.

8. Use one tablespoon olive oil to brush the baking dish.

9. Take the bag from the boiling water when the timer goes off.

10. Pick the sunchokes and hold the dry ones from the package. Let them cool.

11. Crush each one with the palm of your hand when they are about half-inch thick and when sunchokes are easy enough to manage.

12. Position the sunchokes and drizzle with the leftover two tablespoons of olive oil on the baking dish and season with pepper and salt.

13. Roast sunchokes, tossing half-way back, 20 to 25 minutes until the sides are crispy and fresh.

14. Toss the almonds on the tops of the sunchokes, then proceed to roast for 2 minutes till the almonds are brown.

15. Move sunchokes and seasoning with chives onto a serving tray. Serve immediately.

31. TURMERIC AND DILL PICKLED CAULIFLOWER

Cal.: 320 | Fat: 27g | Protein: 14g

Preparation Time: 13 minutes
Cooking Time: 6 hours 10 minutes
Servings: 4

Ingredients

A few sprigs dill
1 tablespoon black peppercorns
1 tablespoon salt
1 (thumb-sized piece) turmeric (sliced)
1 cup water
¼ cup sugar
4 cups cauliflower florets
1 cup white wine vinegar

Directions

1. Preheat the Sous Vide machine to 140°F/60°C.

2. In a pan, combine the water, salt, vinegar, black peppercorn, sugar and turmeric.

3. Simmer to remove the sugar.

4. Load the florets and dill sprigs of cauliflower into pureeing pots.

---

5. Through the pots, pour the pickling liquid.

6. Keep the jars sealed.

7. Cook for 3 hours.

8. Carry out the pot of water and leave overnight on your kitchen table.

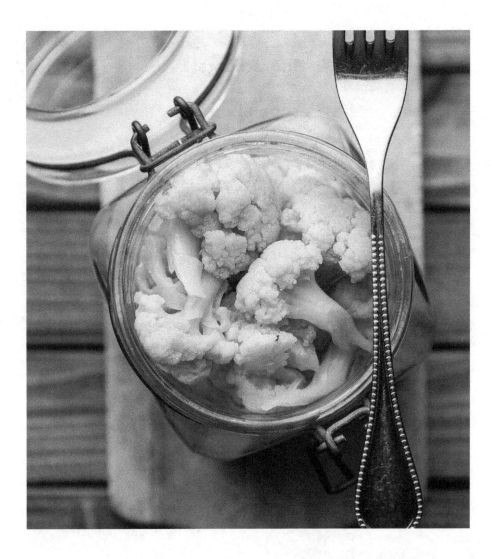

32. DOENJANG-SPICED EGGPLANT

Cal.: 243 | Fat: 26g | Protein: 14g

Preparation Time: 9 minutes
Cooking Time: 1 hour 35 minutes
Servings: 2

Ingredients

1 tablespoon brown sugar
1 tablespoon sesame seeds
2 tablespoons Doenjang paste
2 tablespoons soy sauce
¼ cup peanut oil
4 pieces Thai eggplants (cut into wedges)

Directions

1. In a cup, whisk together the Doenjang mixture, peanut oil, soya sauce and sugar.

2. In the cup, add the eggplants and mix to fill uniformly.

3. In a Sous Vide pack, position the eggplants and sauces.

4. Set your Sous Vide machine to 185°F/85°C, simmer for 45 minutes.

5. Wash the wedges of the eggplant from the water for frying.

6. Cook in a frying skillet with the eggplants.

7. While eating, fill with sesame seeds.

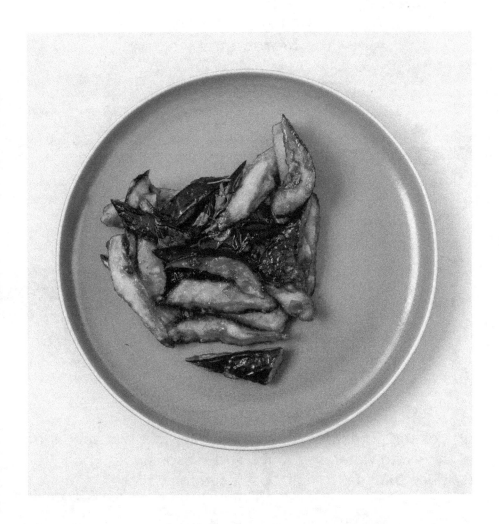

33. TOMATO SUSHI

Cal.: 480 | Fat: 36g | Protein: 19g

Preparation Time: 8 minutes
Cooking Time: 16 hours
Servings: 12

Ingredients

For the Tomatoes:
¼ Teaspoon salt
1 cup water
3 pieces Roma tomatoes
1 tablespoon soy sauce
3 sheets nori
For the Sushi Rice:
2 tablespoons sugar
¼ teaspoon salt
¼ cup rice vinegar
1.5 cups water
1 cup (uncooked) glutinous white rice

Directions

1. For the Tomatoes: In a frying pan, mix two sheets of nori with water, soy sauce and seasoning and boil. Reduce the heat to half. Just leave to cool.

2. Pick each tomato and gently cut an "X" with a matching knife with one end.

3. Place the tomatoes for 30 seconds to a few minutes in boiling water.

4. Place the tomatoes in an iced bath.

5. Peel, half, and toss the tomatoes down.

6. During the nori decrease (sauce thickening process), marinate the tomatoes for 4 hours.

7. Place the tomatoes in a Sous Vide pocket with the marinade and bake at 140°F/60°Cfor 4 hours.

8. For rice sushi: In a casserole dish, boil the vinegar, salt and sugar until the sugar is fully dissolved.

9. Under cold water, drain the glutinous rice.

10. Combine a bowl of rice and water. Just get it to a boil.

11. Decrease the heat to a simmer after boiling, then bring to boil for 15 minutes.

12. Pour the combination of vinegar and sugar over the rice and stir.

13. Assembling: Shape the rice into sushi pieces with your fingertips.

14. Top each section of tomato sushi rice and cover it with a nori bar.

34. SMOKY BBQ BUTTER CORN

Cal.: 242 | Fat: 28g | Protein: 9g

Preparation Time: 11 minutes
Cooking Time: 1 hour 5 minutes
Servings: 3

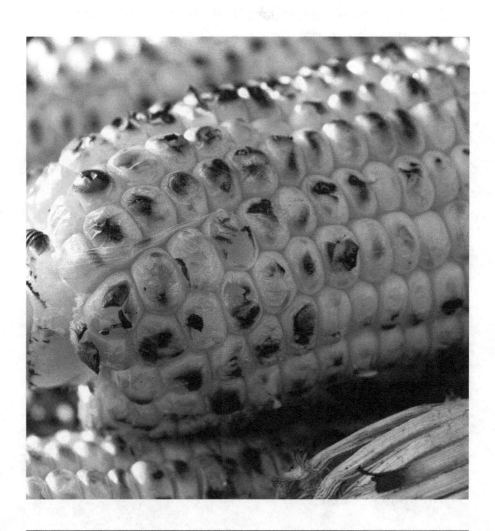

Ingredients

2 tablespoons smoky BBQ spice blend
½ stick butter.
3 ears corn husked (ends trimmed)

Directions

1. Add the melted butter and BBQ seasoning together.

2. Rub corn with BBQ butter across.

3. In a Sous Vide jar, place the buttered corn and the leftover butter.

4. Heat at 183°F/84°C for thirty minutes.

5. Serve!

35. CHILI-GARLIC TOFU

Cal.: 421 | Fat: 32g | Protein: 19g

Preparation Time: 9 minutes
Cooking Time: 8 hours 10 minutes
Servings: 4

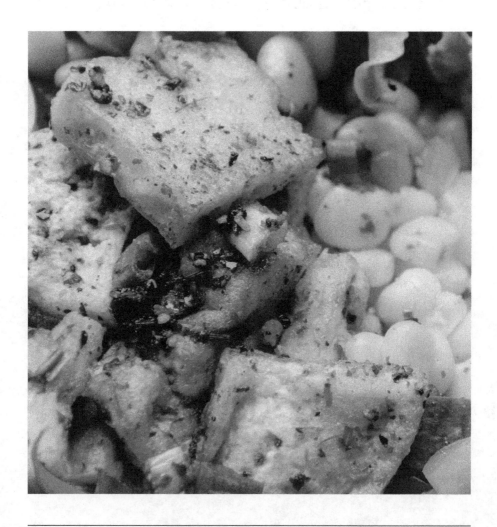

Ingredients

¼ Cup sesame oil
2 tablespoons chili-garlic (paste)
1 block firm tofu (cut into slices)
½ cup brown sugar
¼ cup soy sauce

Directions

1. Hot skillet-fry pieces of tofu until they are nicely browned.

2. In a pan, mix all the remaining ingredients.

3. Toss in the sauce with the tofu pieces.

4. In a Sous Vide packet, bring the tofu along with the sauce.

5. Heat at 180°F/82°C for 4 hours.

6. Serve!

36. CRISP CORN WITH BUTTER AND FRESH HERBS

Cal.: 179 | Fat: 20g | Protein: 11g

Preparation Time: 18 minutes
Cooking Time: 30 minutes
Servings: 4

Ingredients

2.8g black pepper
Fresh herbs
57g butter
5 fresh thyme, sprigs
60 ml of olive oil
383g corn
2.8g salt
3 garlic cloves (peeled)

Directions

1. Preheat the Sous Vide Machine to 194 °F / 90 °C.

2. On the grill, pour oil into a pan. Add sliced garlic cloves. Keep frying on medium-high heat, spooning oil on the garlic until the cloves become brown and roasted for about 10 minutes.

3. Move the oil and leave to cool down for 15 minutes in a shallow dish.

4. Using your fingertips, pull at the corn packaging the blob and linen to extract them from the sides of the corn. A few at a time, horizontally tilt each cob over a bowl. Then, remove corn from cob by slicing directly downwards with a sharp knife.

5. Transfer the corn kernels to the vacuum sealer bag and add salt, butter, roasted garlic, and thyme.

6. Seal the bag. Lower the vacuum-sealed bag into the water. If the bag floats, use tongs to weigh it down.

7. Cook for 20 minutes. Transfer corn to a serving dish and garnish with pepper, infused garlic oil, fresh herbs, edible flowers, or whatever you like.

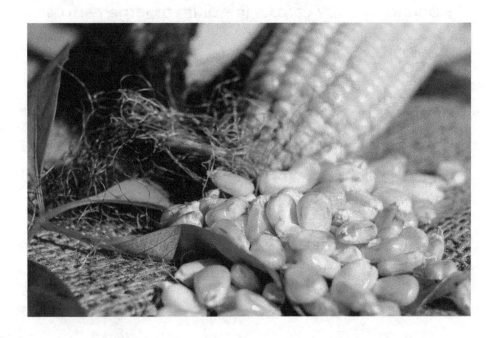

37. GLAZED CARROTS

Cal.: 70 | Fat: 11g | Protein: 6g

Preparation Time: 9 minutes
Cooking Time: 1 hour
Servings: 6

Ingredients

Freshly ground black pepper
1 tablespoon chopped parsley
1 tablespoon granulated sugar
2 tablespoons unsalted butter
Kosher salt
1 pound of baby carrots (medium to large carrots)

Directions

1. Preheat the Sous Vide machine to 183°F/84°C.

2. In a vacuum bag, put the vegetables, butter, sugar, and 1 tablespoon kosher salt and seal as instructed by the supplier.

3. In boiling water, boil the carrot until absolutely tender, for around 1 hour.

4. At this stage, carrots can be kept for up to 1 week in the refrigerator.

5. Load the entire contents of the package into a high-bottomed 12-inch oven and bake over medium temperature, stirring vigorously for about 2 minutes, until the liquid is reduced to a glossy glaze.

6. Season with salt to taste, whisk in the parsley, and prepare.

7. If glaze cracks and becomes greasy, apply water about 1 tablespoon at a time, shake the pot to re-form coating.

38. FRENCH FRIES

Cal.: 85 | Fat: 2g | Protein: 9g

Preparation Time: 11 minutes
Cooking Time: 55 minutes
Servings: 4

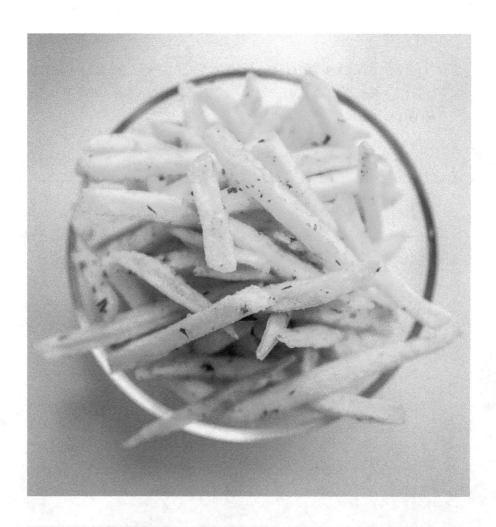

Ingredients

Vegetable oil for frying
Salt to taste
¼ teaspoon sugar
¼ teaspoon baking soda
500 grams of potatoes, peeled.
½ tablespoon salt
½ cup water

Directions

1. Combine the water, sugar, salt, and baking soda together.

2. Place potatoes in the pocket with the salted water.

3. Cook in the Sous Vide at 194°F/90°C for 15 minutes.

4. Let potatoes dry.

5. Fry for 7 minutes at 266°F/130°C.

6. Let it soak and cool.

7. Fry for 2 minutes at 374°F/190°C.

39. THYME-INFUSED MUSHROOMS

Cal.: 125 | Fat: 20g | Protein: 22g

Preparation Time: 9 minutes
Cooking Time: 45 minutes
Servings: 4

Ingredients

2 large garlic cloves, sliced
Salt to taste
1 pinch freshly, ground black, pepper
2 tablespoons olive oil
1 tablespoon chopped, fresh, flat-leaf parsley
1 tablespoon olive oil
1 tablespoon chopped, fresh thyme
1 pound of sliced mushrooms

Directions

1. In a plastic storage jar, mix the mushrooms, parsley, thyme and one tablespoon of olive oil.

2. To spread the seasonings, apply fresh peppers and lift.

3. To clear the air and close the container, please use a vacuum sealer.

4. Preheat the Sous Vide machine to 175°F/79°C.

5. Lower the sealable bag and drench it in the water. Set a 30-minute timer.

6. Use stainless steel tweezers to keep the package in position if you don't have a Sous Vide stand.

7. In the meantime, prepare 2 tablespoons of olive oil on medium heat in a casserole dish and insert minced garlic.

8. To infuse the oil, cook it for 10 minutes.

9. Remove from the heat until the mushrooms are fully cooked.

10. When the mushrooms are fully cooked, on medium-high heat, heat the garlic oil.

11. Use a rubber spatula to pick the mushrooms out of the package and sauté them in garlic oil for 3 minutes. Season with salt and pepper.

40. FLAN

Cal.: 120 | Fat: 2g | Protein: 9g

Preparation Time: 8 minutes
Cooking Time: 1 hour 35 minutes
Servings: 8

Ingredients

3 large eggs
1 tablespoon vanilla extract
1 can (sweetened) condensed milk
1 can evaporated milk
¾ cup white sugar
4-ounce jars with lids

Directions

1. In a wide heat-proof bowl full of water, put a Sous Vide cook within.

2. Preheat medium 179°F/81°C. water tank.

3. Melt the sugar in a small saucepan for around 5 minutes, until golden brown.

4. Load 8 4-ounce Mason jars of hot molten sugar, enough to hit the end of each.

---

5. In a separate cup, combine the condensed milk, evaporated milk, eggs and vanilla extract separately.

6. Add to the bottles and seal.

7. In the water bath, put the jars and set a timer for 1one hour.

8. Replace the boiling water jars. Let cool for about 20 minutes, before safe to touch.

9. Uncover the jars and run along the edges of the flan with a thin rubber spatula.

10. Use a plate to cover each flan; turn the side and shake thoroughly.

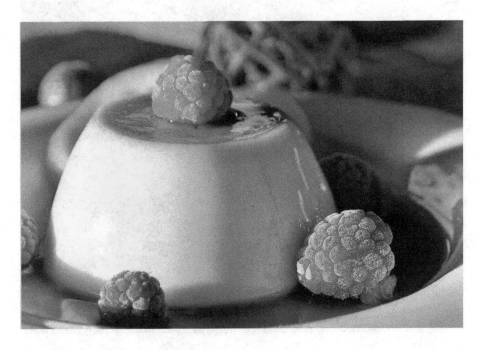

41. SPICY EGGPLANT

Cal.: 65 | Fat: 1.5g | Protein: 2.8g

Preparation Time: 10 minutes
Cooking Time: 25 minutes
Servings: 4

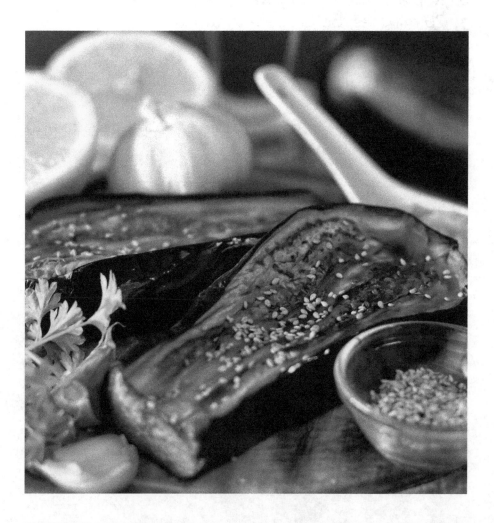

Ingredients

1-pound eggplants, sliced
¼ cup lemon juice
2 tablespoons olive oil
½ teaspoon hot paprika
1 red chili pepper, minced.
1 tablespoon chili powder
A pinch of salt and black pepper

Directions

1. In a large bag, mix the eggplants with the lemon juice, oil and the other ingredients, seal the bag, immerse in the water bath, cook at 170°F/76°C. for 25 minutes, divide the mix between plates and serve.

2. Use a plate to cover each flan; turn the side and shake thoroughly.

42. PESTO TOMATO MIX

Cal.: 25 | Fat: 1.9g | Protein: 1.4g

Preparation Time: 10 minutes
Cooking Time: 20 minutes
Servings: 4

Ingredients

1 pound cherry tomatoes, halved.
2 tablespoons olive oil
2 tablespoons basil pesto
½ teaspoon sweet paprika
1 teaspoon garlic, minced.
A pinch of salt and black pepper
1 tablespoon chives, chopped.

Directions

1. In a bag, mix the tomatoes with the pesto, oil and the other ingredients, seal the bag, cook in the water bath at 167°F/75°C for 20 minutes, divide the mix between plates and serve.

43. CABBAGE SAUTÉ

Cal.: 36 | Fat: 1.4g | Protein: 2g

Preparation Time: 10 minutes
Cooking Time: 25 minutes
Servings: 4

Ingredients

1-pound red cabbage, shredded
1 tablespoon lime juice
2 tablespoons olive oil
1 teaspoon sweet paprika
A pinch of salt and black pepper
¼ cup chicken stock
1 tablespoon dill, chopped.

Directions

1. In a bag, mix the cabbage with the lime juice, oil and the other ingredients, seal the bag, cook in the water bath at 170°F/76°C for 25 minutes, divide the mix between plates and serve.

44. PAPRIKA OKRA

Cal.: 26 | Fat: 1.2g | Protein: 1.4g

Preparation Time: 10 minutes
Cooking Time: 25 minutes
Servings: 4

Ingredients

2 cups okra
1 teaspoon sweet paprika
1 tablespoon olive oil
1 tablespoon lemon juice
A pinch of salt and black pepper
1 tablespoon balsamic vinegar
1 tablespoon chives, chopped.

Directions

1. In a bag, mix the okra with the lemon juice, paprika and the other ingredients, seal the bag, cook in the water bath at 160°F/71°C for 25 minutes, divide the mix between plates and serve.

45. ZUCCHINI AND TOMATO MIX

Cal.: 41 | Fat: 1.2g | Protein: 2.4g

Preparation Time: 10 minutes
Cooking Time: 30 minutes
Servings: 4

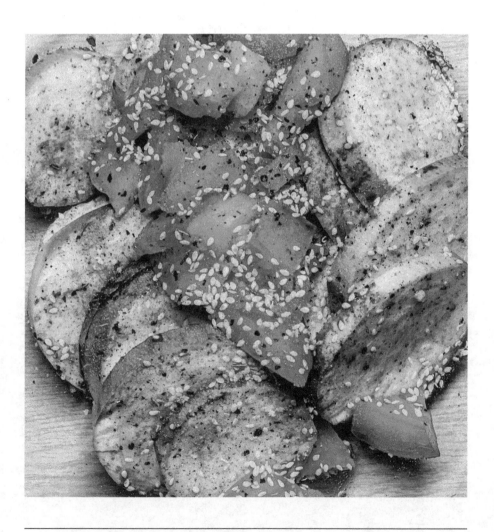

Ingredients

2 cups zucchinis, sliced.
1 cup cherry tomatoes, halved.
2 tablespoons olive oil
2 tablespoons balsamic vinegar
A pinch of salt and black pepper
2 tablespoons parsley, chopped.

Directions

1. In a bag, mix the zucchinis with the tomatoes and the other ingredients, seal the bag, immerse in the water bath, cook at 160°F/71°C for 30 minutes, divide the mix between plates and serve.

46. CHILI COLLARD GREENS

Cal.: 151 | Fat: 12.2g | Protein: 4g

Preparation Time: 10 minutes
Cooking Time: 20 minutes
Servings: 4

Ingredients

1 pound collard greens, trimmed.
2 tablespoons balsamic vinegar
½ teaspoon chili powder
1 red chili pepper, minced.
2 tablespoons olive oil
1 tablespoon sweet paprika
A pinch of salt and black pepper
1 tablespoon cilantro, chopped.

Directions

1. In a bag, mix the collard greens with the vinegar, chili powder and the other ingredients, seal the bag, cook in the water bath at 160°F/71°C for 20 minutes, divide the mix between plates and serve. the mix between plates and serve.

47. BEET AND RADISH MIX

Cal.: 61 | Fat: 1.3g | Protein: 3.2g

Preparation Time: 10 minutes
Cooking Time: 35 minutes
Servings: 4

Ingredients

1-pound radishes, halved
½ pound beets, peeled and cut into wedges.
2 tablespoons olive oil
2 tablespoons balsamic vinegar
1 tablespoon chives, chopped.
A pinch of salt and black pepper

Directions

1. In a bag, mix the radishes with the beets, oil and the rest of the ingredients, seal the bag, cook in the water oven at 167°F/75°C for 35 minutes, divide the mix between plates and serve.

48. CILANTRO HOT ARTICHOKES

Cal.: 141 | Fat: 1.5g | Protein: 7.3g

Preparation Time: 10 minutes
Cooking Time: 30 minutes
Servings: 4

Ingredients

½ cup canned artichoke hearts, drained and
chopped (you can use fresh artichokes as well).
2 red chilies, minced.
½ teaspoon hot paprika
1 tablespoon cilantro, chopped.
2 tablespoons olive oil
2 tablespoons balsamic vinegar
A pinch of red pepper flakes, crushed.
A pinch of salt and black pepper

Directions

1. In a large bag, mix the artichoke hearts with the chilies and the other ingredients, seal the bag, cook in the water bath at 170°F/76°C. for 30 minutes, divide the mix between plates and serve. the mix between plates and serve.

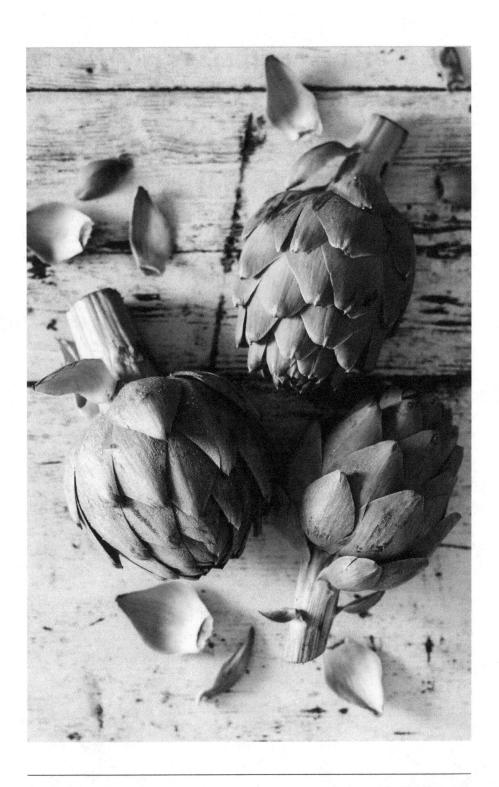

49. TOFU MARINATED WITH HARISSA AND KALE

Cal.: 321 | Fat: 11g | Protein: 20g

Preparation Time: 15 minutes
Cooking Time: from 2 to 3 hours
Servings: 4

Ingredients

For the Sous Vide Tofu
1 package firm or extra-firm tofu, about 14 ounces
3 tablespoons harissa or other chile-garlic sauce
1 tablespoon soy sauce
For the Kale
1 tablespoon sesame oil
3 cups coarsely chopped kale
3 cloves garlic, minced
2 tablespoons minced ginger
2 tablespoons soy sauce
1 tablespoon rice wine vinegar
To Assemble
1 cup cooked farro
1 1/2 cups cooked lentils
1/2 cup roasted red peppers
1/4 cup chopped fresh basil leaves

Directions

1. Preheat your sous vide to 180°F (82.2°C).

2. Drain the tofu and cut into slabs, 3/4" to 1" thick. Place the slabs on paper towels, cover with paper towels some light weight. Let it rest for 30 minutes.

3. Mix the harissa and soy sauce. Remove the cover from the tofu and brush with the mixture. Place the tofu in a sous vide bag and seal it. Place the bag in the water bath and cook for 2 to 3 hours.

4. To prepare the Kale: In a pan, using medium heat, warm the sesame oil. Add the kale, garlic, ginger, soy sauce and vinegar. Cover the pan and let cook until the kale is tender. It should take around 20/30 minutes.

5. To Assemble the dish: Remove the bag from the water bath, extract the tofu and dry thoroughly using paper towels. Sear the tofu; you can do ut using a torch, a broiler or a pan. When the tofu's sourface is slightly brown, remove from the heat and cut into bite-sized chunks.

6. Place the farro and lentils in a bowl and top with the kale and its juices. Add the tofu and the roasted red peppers. Sprinkle with the basil then serve.

50. STUFFED CAULIFLOWER

Cal.: 143 | Fat: 2.4g | Protein: 3.2g

Preparation Time: 20 minutes
Cooking Time: 1 hour 10 minutes
Servings: 4-6

Ingredients

For the cauliflower:
1 cauliflower – destalked and core removed.
100ml water
5g salt
1 g yellow mustard seeds.
2 g fennel seeds
2g coriander seeds

For the stuffing:
100g of tinned chickpeas cooked
80g tinned fava beans cooked
20g juice from the fava bean tin
20g chickpea water
¼ lemon zest
10g chopped cranberry
20g chopped cashew nuts
20 g chopped chickpea and fava beans.
10ml red wine vinegar
¼ lemon juice

Directions

1. Preheat the sous vide to 180°F (82°C)

2. Seal a sous vide bag with the cauliflower, water, salt, mustard seeds, fennel seeds, and coriander seeds. Cooking time is 20-30 minutes.

3. Remove from the water bath and set aside to cool.

4. Blend the chickpeas, fava beans, juice, chickpea water, and lemon zest until the mixture is semi-smooth.

5. Then add cranberries, cashew nuts, chopped chickpea and fava beans, red wine vinegar, and lemon juice. Season to taste.

6. Pre-heat your oven to 390°F (200°C).

7. Take the cauliflower out of the pouch and set it aside.

8. Squeeze the mixture in between the cauliflower florets with a spoon or piping bag, then bake for 30-45 minutes, until golden.

TEMPERATURE CHARTS

🥕 VEGETABLES	°F🌡 TEMPERA-TURE	⏱ TIME
Vegetables, root (carrots, potato, parsnips, beets, celery root, turnips)	183 °F	3 hours
Vegetables, tender (asparagus, broccoli, cauliflower, fennel, onions, pumpkin, eggplant, green beans, corn)	183 °F	1 hour
Vegetables, greens (kale, spinach, collard greens, Swiss chard)	183 °F	3 min.

🍐 FRUITS	°F🌡 TEMPERA-TURE	⏱ TIME
Fruit, firm (apple, pear)	183 °F	45 min.
Fruit, for purée	185 °F	30 min.
Fruit, berries for topping desserts (blueberries, blackberries, raspberries, strawberries, cranberries)	154 °F	30 min.

WHAT TEMPERATURE SHOULD BE USED?

The rule of thumb is that the thicker the piece, the longer it should cook. Higher temperatures shorten the cooking time. Lower temperatures may take longer.

	TEMPERA-TURE	MIN COOK-ING TIME	MAX COOK-ING TIME
GREEN VEGETABLES			
Rare	183°F (84°C)	¼ hour	¾ hour
ROOTS			
Rare	183°F (84°C)	1 hour	3 hours
FRUITS			
Warm	154°F (68°C)	1¾ hour	2½ hour
Soft Fruits	185°F (85°C)	½ hour	1½ hour

COOKING CONVERSION

TEMPERATURE CONVERSIONS	
CELSIUS	**FAHRENHEIT**
54.5°C	130°F
60.0°C	140°F
65.5°C	150°F
71.1°C	160°F
76.6°C	170°F
82.2°C	180°F
87.8°C	190°F
93.3°C	200°F
100°C	212°F

WEIGHT COVERSION	
½ oz.	15g
1 oz.	30g
2 oz.	60g
3 oz.	85g
4 oz.	110g
5 oz.	140g
6 oz.	170g
7 oz.	200g
8 oz.	225g
9 oz.	255g
10 oz.	280g
11 oz.	310g
12 oz.	340g
13 oz.	370g
14 oz.	400g
15 oz.	425g
1 lb.	450g

LIQUID VOLUME CONVERSION		
CUPS / TABLE-SPOONS	**FL. OUNCES**	**MILLILITERS**
1 cup	8 fl. Oz.	240 ml
¾ cup	6 fl. Oz.	180 ml
2/3 cup	5 fl. Oz.	150 ml
½ cup	4 fl. Oz.	120 ml
1/3 cup	2 ½ fl. Oz.	75 ml
¼ cup	2 fl. Oz.	60 ml
1/8 cup	1 fl. Oz.	30 ml
1 tablespoon	½ fl. Oz.	15 ml

TEASPOON (tsp.) / TABLESPOON (Tbsp.)	**MILLILITERS**
1 tsp.	5ml
2 tsp.	10ml
1 Tbsp.	15ml
2 Tbsp.	30ml
3 Tbsp.	45ml
4 Tbsp.	60ml
5 Tbsp.	75ml
6 Tbsp.	90ml
7 Tbsp.	105ml

LIQUID VOLUME MEASUREMENTS			
TABLE-SPOONS	TEASPOONS	FLUID OUNCES	CUPS
16	48	8 fl. Oz.	1
12	36	6 fl. Oz.	¾
8	24	4 fl. Oz.	½
5 ½	16	2 2/3 fl. Oz.	1/3
4	12	2 fl. Oz.	¼
1	3	0.5 fl. Oz.	1/16

RECIPE INDEX

CPSIA information can be obtained
at www.ICGtesting.com
Printed in the USA
BVHW090221110521
606943BV00004B/825